Air Fryer Grill Cookbook for Beginners

A Transforming Guide on The Best Quick and Tasty, Time-Saving, Easy and Mouth-Watering Indoor Grill and Griddle Recipes for Fast & Healthy Meals for Everyday Cooking

Paty Breads

TABLE OF CONTENTS

Introduction

The Power Air Fryer Grill may be a sophisticated machine imbued with modern technology for cooking healthy and luxurious meals quickly and as fast as possible. It's a multi-functional Air Fryer plus grill amid eight cook programs and intrinsic cooking presets. With the rapid air technology, heated air at 450°F circulates and cooks your meals 40% faster than ordinary/traditional cooking methods.

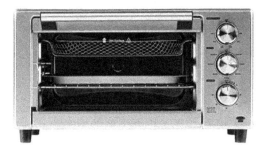

The Power Air Fryer Grill cuts calories in your meals by 70% due to the small quantity of oil required to grill, fry, and bake. It also saves time, counter space, and even the environment since it works via electricity.

Components and Functions of Power Air Fryer Grill

The Power Air Fryer Grill may be a box-like appliance comprising eight cooking/preset programs and straightforward work commands. The components and functions are as follows:

- The central unit may be a chrome steel construct that houses the component, instrument panel, and cooking accessories (pans, trays, and racks) through the three available tray ports.
- The tempered glass door keeps the warmth in and allows for even circulation of the recent air. Open and shut the door with the handle attached to avoid burns from the heated glass.
- The chrome steel drip tray placed below the component collects fluids and oils in cooking; if the drip tray is absent while cooking, it causes smoke and damaged heating coils.

- The grill plate is used to grill meat, burgers, vegetables, and more.
- The pizza rack is used to roast, toast bread & bagel, make pizza, and grill.
- The baking pan and the crisper tray are used to broil and make food without oil content.
- The instrument panel comprises knobs and buttons to regulate and adjust the time, temperature, and cooking programs. The preset programs are: air fry, grill, air fry/grill, rotisserie, toast/bagel, and pizza/bake, broil, and reheat.

How Power Air Fryer Grill Functions

- Set up your unit on a good, flat surface, preferably a cool countertop, far away from other appliances, and in a well-ventilated room. Plug the cord into a wall plug.
- Place the drip tray correctly at the unit's bottom and insert the proper accessory to make the food.
- Arrange the ingredients inside the unit.
- Select the specified cook program with the function knob.
- Select the temperature and time with the temperature/darkness control knob and, therefore, the time control knob. The facility light then comes on.
- The power light darkens, and the timer sounds once the cooking process ends. Note that foods cooked for fewer than 20 minutes don't activate the timer sound. Turn all knobs to the offsetting before opening the unit to get food.

Maintenance, Cleaning, and Tips

Proper and regular maintenance is crucial to machinery's long lifetime, and therefore the Power Air Fryer Grill isn't an exception.

- When unpacking for the first time, read all instructions and warnings, remove all labels, and wash all accessories with warm water and soap by hand. Preheat to reduce the producer's oil coat. Make sure you wipe off the melted oil with a moist rag before use.
- All accessories are dishwasher safe. Wash with soap and water. Most units must not be soaked or dipped in water but gently wiped inside and out first with a hot/soapy damp/soft rag then rinsed with a classic moist rag. Ensure it's completely dry before you turning it on.
- Wear protective gloves or oven mitts when handling any part of the Air Fryer grill to avoid burns.
- The Air Fryer grill is for indoor use only. Connect only to direct power sources, sort of wall plug, and never an extension box to avoid tripping accidents.
- The more the number of food, the longer it takes to cook and the other way around.
- You may use an oven dish or baking tin for filled foods like soups by placing it on the rack.
- Use parchment paper on the Air Fryer rack and drip pan to stop smoke as grease drops on the heating coils.
- Judiciously study the user manual of your appliance to stop eventualities and cure them.

Chapter 1:

Breakfast Recipes

1. Breakfast Egg Tomato

Preparation time: 10 minutes.

Cooking time: 24 minutes.

Servings: 2

Ingredients:

- 2 eggs

- 2 large fresh tomatoes

- 1 teaspoon fresh parsley

- Pepper to taste

- Salt to taste

Directions:

1. Preheat the Air Fryer to 325°F.

2. Cut off the top of a tomato and spoon out the tomato innards.

3. Break the egg in each tomato and place it in the Air Fryer basket and cook for 24 minutes.

4. Season with parsley, pepper, and salt.

5. Serve and enjoy!

Nutrition:

- **Calories:** 95

- **Fat:** 5g

- **Carbohydrates:** 7.5g

- **Sugar:** 5.1g

- **Protein:** 7g

- **Cholesterol:** 164mg

2. Mushroom Leek Frittata

Preparation time: 10 minutes.

Cooking time: 32 minutes.

Servings: 4

Ingredients:

- 6 eggs

- 6 ounces mushrooms, sliced

- 1 cup leeks, sliced

- Salt to taste

Directions:

1. Preheat the Air Fryer to 325°F.

2. Heat another pan over medium heat. Spray pan with cooking spray.

3. Add mushrooms, leeks, and salt in a pan, sauté for 6 minutes.

4. Break eggs in a bowl and whisk well.

5. Transfer sautéed mushroom and leek mixture into the prepared baking dish.

6. Pour egg over mushroom mixture.

7. Put it in the Air Fryer, then cook for 32 minutes.

8. Serve and enjoy!

Nutrition:

- **Calories:** 116

- **Fat:** 7g

- **Carbohydrates:** 5.1g

- **Sugar:** 2.1g

- **Protein:** 10g

- **Cholesterol:** 245mg

3. Wild Blueberry Bagels

Preparation time: 11 minutes.

Cooking time: 5 minutes.

Servings: 1

Ingredients:

- 1 bagel

- 1 tablespoon low-fat cream cheese

- 2 tablespoons frozen wild blueberries

- 1/4 teaspoon cinnamon

Directions:

1. Preheat the Power Air Fryer Grill to 190°C or 375°F.

2. Toast the bagel for 3–5 minutes.

3. Spread cream cheese; add blueberry toppings, and cinnamon.

Nutrition:

- **Calories:** 155 **Protein:** 6g **Fat:** 3.5g

4. Southwestern Waffles

Preparation time: 8 minutes.

Cooking time: 6 minutes.

Servings: 4

Ingredients:

- 1 egg, fried

- 1/4 avocado, chopped

- 1 frozen waffle

- 1 tablespoon salsa

Directions:

1. Preheat the Power Air Fryer Grill to 200°C or 400°F.

2. Bake the waffles for 5–7 minutes.

3. Add avocado, fried eggs, and fresh salsa as toppings.

Nutrition:

- **Calories:** 207 **Protein:** 9g **Fat:** 12g

5. Pumpkin Spice Bagels

Preparation time: 18 minutes.

Cooking time: 12 minutes.

Servings: 2

Ingredients:

- 1 egg

- 1 cup flour

- 1/2 teaspoon pumpkin spice

- 1/2 cup Greek yogurt

Directions

1. Make a dough with flour, pie spice, yogurt, and pumpkin in a stand mixer.

2. Shape the dough into a few ropes and make bagels.

3. Apply egg and water mixture over the bagels.

4. Preheat the Power Air Fryer Grill to 190°C or 375°F and bake

   for 20–25 minutes.

Nutrition

- **Calories:** 183

- **Protein:** 9.4g

- **Fat:** 2g

6. Bacon, Egg and Cheese Breakfast Hash

Preparation time: 12 minutes.

Cooking time: 35 minutes.

Servings: 4

Ingredients:

- 2 slices of bacon

- 4 tiny potatoes

- 1/4 tomato

- 1 egg

- 1/4 cup of shredded cheese

Directions:

1. Preheat the Power Air Fryer Grill to 200°C or 400°F on bake mode. Set bits of bacon on a double-layer tin foil.

2. Cut the vegetables to put over the bacon. Crack an egg over it.

3. Shape the tin foil into a bowl and cook it in the Power Air Fryer Grill at 177°C or 350°F for 15–20 minutes. Put some shredded cheese on top.

Nutrition:

- **Calories:** 150.5

- **Protein:** 6g

- **Fat:** 6g

7. Southwestern Hash with Eggs

Preparation time: 25 minutes.

Cooking time: 45 minutes.

Servings: 4

Ingredients:

- 1–1/2 pound pork steak 1 teaspoon vegetable oil

- 1 large potato, peeled and cubed

- 1 medium-sized onion, chopped

- 1 garlic clove, minced

- 1/2 cup green pepper, chopped

- 1 can diced tomatoes and green chilies

- 1 beef bouillon cube

- 1/2 teaspoon ground cumin

- 1/2 teaspoon salt

- 1/4 teaspoon pepper

- 1/8 teaspoon cayenne pepper

- 4 eggs

- 3/4 cup shredded Cheddar cheese

- 4 corn tortillas (6 inches)

Directions:

1. Cook pork in oil until brown and add potato, onion, garlic, green pepper. Cook for 4 minutes.

2. Stir in tomatoes, bouillon, cumin, salt, pepper, and cayenne. Cook over low heat until potatoes become tender.

3. Make four wells inside the hash and crack eggs into them.

4. Bake it in the Power Air Fryer Grill uncovered for 10–12 minutes at 177°C or 350°F and scatter some cheese over it.

5. Serve over tortillas.

Nutrition:

- **Calories:** 520 **Protein:** 49g **Fat:** 23g

Chapter 2:

Meat Recipes

8. Pork Satay

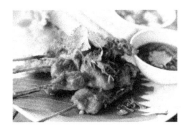

Preparation time: 15 minutes.

Cooking time: 9–14 minutes. **Servings:** 4

Ingredients:

- 1(1-pound) pork tenderloin, cut into 1½-inch cubes

- ¼ cup minced onion

- 2 garlic cloves, minced

- 1 jalapeno pepper, minced

- 2 tablespoons freshly squeezed lime juice

- 2 tablespoons coconut milk

- 2 tablespoons unsalted peanut butter

- 2 teaspoons curry powder

Directions:

1. In a medium bowl, mix the pork, onion, garlic, jalapeno, lime juice, coconut milk, peanut butter, and curry powder until well combined. Let stand for 10 minutes at room temperature.

2. With a slotted spoon, remove the pork from the marinade. Reserve the marinade.

3. Thread the pork onto about 8 bamboo or metal skewers. Grill for 9 to 14 minutes, brushing once with the reserved marinade until the pork reaches at least 145°F on a meat thermometer. Discard any remaining marinade. Serve immediately.

Nutrition: Calories: 194 **Fat:** 7g **Protein:** 25g

9. Pork Burgers with Red Cabbage Salad

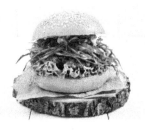

Preparation time: 20 minutes.

Cooking time: 7–9 minutes.

Servings: 4

Ingredients:

- ½ cup Greek yogurt

- 2 tablespoons low-sodium mustard, divided

- 1 tablespoon lemon juice

- ¼ cup sliced red cabbage

- ¼ cup grated carrots

- 1-pound lean ground pork

- ½ teaspoon paprika

- 1 cup mixed baby lettuce greens

- 2 small tomatoes, sliced

- 8 small low-sodium whole-wheat sandwich buns, cut in half

Directions:

1. In a small bowl, combine the yogurt, 1 tablespoon of mustard, lemon juice, cabbage, and carrots mix and refrigerate.

2. In a medium bowl, combine the pork, the remaining 1 tablespoon of mustard, and paprika. Form into 8 small patties.

3. Put the sliders into the Air Fryer basket. Grill for 7 to 9 minutes, or until the sliders register 165°F as tested with a meat thermometer.

4. Assemble the burgers by placing some of the lettuce greens on a bun bottom. Top with a tomato slice, the burgers, and the cabbage mixture. Add the bun top and serve immediately.

Nutrition:

- **Calories:** 472 **Fat:** 15g **Protein:** 35g

10. Crispy Mustard Pork Tenderloin

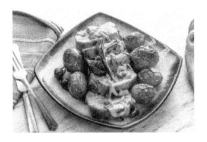

Preparation time: 10 minutes.

Cooking time: 12–16 minutes.

Servings: 4

Ingredients:

- 3 tablespoons low-sodium grainy mustard

- 2 teaspoons olive oil

- ¼ teaspoon dry mustard powder

- 1(1-pound) pork tenderloin, silver skin, and excess fat trimmed

  and discarded

- 2 slices low-sodium whole-wheat bread, crumbled

- ¼ cup ground walnuts

- 2 tablespoons cornstarch

Directions:

1. In a small bowl, stir together the mustard, olive oil, and mustard powder. Spread this mixture over the pork.

2. On a plate, mix the breadcrumbs, walnuts, and cornstarch. Dip the mustard-coated pork into the crumb mixture to coat.

3. Air-fry the pork for 12 to 16 minutes or until it registers at least 145°F on a meat thermometer. Slice to serve.

Nutrition:

- **Calories:** 239

- **Fat:** 9g

- **Protein:** 26g

11. Apple Pork Tenderloin

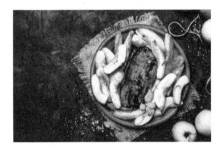

Preparation time: 10 minutes.

Cooking time: 14–19 minutes.

Servings: 4

Ingredients:

- 1(1-pound) pork tenderloin, cut into 4 pieces

- 1 tablespoon apple butter

- 2 teaspoons olive oil

- 2 Granny Smith apples or Jon gold apples, sliced

- 3 celery stalks, sliced

- 1 onion, sliced

- ½ teaspoon dried marjoram

- 1/3 cup apple juice

Directions:

1. Rub each piece of pork with apple butter and olive oil.

2. In a medium metal bowl, mix the pork, apples, celery, onion, marjoram, and apple juice.

3. Place the bowl into the Air Fryer and roast for 14 to 19 minutes, or until the pork reaches at least 145°F on a meat thermometer, and the apples and vegetables are tender. Stir once during cooking. Serve immediately.

Nutrition:

- **Calories:** 213

- **Fat:** 5g

- **Protein:** 24g

12. Apricot Glazed Pork Tenderloins

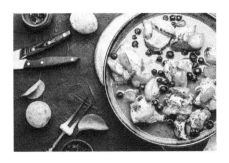

Preparation time: 5 minutes. **Cooking time:** 30 minutes.

Servings: 3

Ingredients:

- 1 teaspoon salt 1/2 teaspoon pepper 1-pound pork tenderloin

- 2 tablespoons minced fresh rosemary or 1 tablespoon dried rosemary, crushed

- 2 tablespoons olive oil, divided

- 3 garlic cloves, minced

Apricot glaze ingredients:

- 1 cup apricot preserves

- 3 garlic cloves, minced

- 4 tablespoons lemon juice

Directions:

1. Mix well pepper, salt, garlic, oil, and rosemary. Brush all over pork. If needed, cut pork crosswise in half to fit in the Air Fryer.

2. Lightly grease the baking pan of the Air Fryer with cooking spray. Add pork.

3. For 3 minutes per side, brown pork in a preheated 390°F Air Fryer.

4. Meanwhile, mix well all glaze Ingredients in a small bowl. Baste pork every 5 minutes.

5. Cook for 20 minutes at 330°F.

6. Serve and enjoy!

Nutrition:

- **Calories:** 281 **Fat:** 9g

- **Protein:** 23g

13. Pork Tenders with Bell Peppers

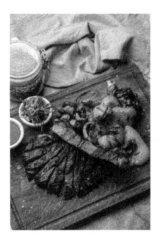

Preparation time: 5 minutes.

Cooking time: 15 minutes. **Servings**: 4

Ingredients:

- 11 ounces pork tenderloin

- 1 bell pepper, in thin strips

- 1 red onion, sliced

- 2 teaspoons. Provencal herbs

- Black pepper to taste

- 1 tablespoon olive oil

- 1/2 tablespoon mustard

Directions:

1. Preheat the power Air Fryer to 390°F.

2. In the oven dish, mix the bell pepper strips with the onion, herbs, and some salt and pepper to taste. Add ½ tablespoon of olive oil to the mixture

3. Cut the pork tenderloin into four pieces and rub it with salt, pepper, and mustard.

4. Thinly coat the pieces with the remaining olive oil and place them upright in the oven dish on top of the pepper mixture.

5. Place the bowl into the power Air Fryer. Set the timer to 15 minutes and roast the meat and the vegetables. Turn the meat and mix the peppers halfway through.

6. Serve with a fresh salad.

Nutrition:

- **Calories:** 273 **Fat:** 10g **Protein:** 20g

14. Barbeque Flavored Pork Ribs

Preparation time: 5 minutes.

Cooking time: 15 minutes.

Servings: 6

Ingredients:

- ¼ cup honey, divided

- ¾ cup BBQ sauce

- 2 tablespoons tomato ketchup

- 1 tablespoon Worcestershire sauce

- 1 tablespoon soy sauce

- ½ teaspoon garlic powder

- Freshly ground white pepper to taste 1(¾) pound pork ribs

Directions:

1. In a large bowl, mix together 3 tablespoons of honey and the

   remaining ingredients, except for pork ribs.

2. Refrigerate to marinate for about 20 minutes.

3. Preheat the power Air Fryer to 355°F.

4. Place the ribs in an Air Fryer basket.

5. Cook for about 13 minutes.

6. Remove the ribs from the power Air Fryer and coat with the remaining honey.

7. Serve hot.

Nutrition:

- **Calories:** 281

- **Fat:** 9g

- **Protein:** 23g

15. Balsamic-Glazed Pork Chops

Preparation time: 5 minutes.

Cooking time: 50 minutes.

Servings: 4

Ingredients:

- ¾ cup balsamic vinegar

- 1(½) tablespoon sugar

- 1 tablespoon butter

- 3 tablespoons olive oil

- 3 tablespoons salt

- 3 pork rib chops

Directions:

1. Place all the ingredients in a bowl and allow the meat to marinate in the fridge for at least 2 hours.

2. Preheat the Air Fryer to 390°F.

3. Place the grill pan accessory in the Air Fryer.

4. Grill the pork chops for 20 minutes, making sure to flip the meat every 10 minutes for even grilling.

5. Meanwhile, pour the balsamic vinegar in a saucepan and allow simmering for at least 10 minutes until the sauce thickens.

6. Brush the meat with the glaze before serving.

Nutrition:

- **Calories:** 274

- **Fat:** 18g

- **Protein:** 17g

16. Rustic Pork Ribs

Preparation time: 5 minutes.

Cooking time: 15 minutes.

Servings: 4

Ingredients:

- 1 rack of pork ribs

- 3 tablespoons dry red wine

- 1 tablespoon soy sauce

- 1/2 teaspoon dried thyme

- 1/2 teaspoon onion powder

- 1/2 teaspoon garlic powder

- 1/2 teaspoon ground black pepper

- 1 teaspoon smoked salt

- 1 tablespoon cornstarch

- 1/2 teaspoon olive oil

Directions:

1. Begin by preheating your power Air Fryer to 390°F. Place all the ingredients in a mixing bowl and let them marinate for at least 1 hour.

2. Cook the marinated ribs for approximately 25 minutes at 390°F.

3. Serve hot.

Nutrition:

- **Calories:** 309

- **Fat:** 11g

- **Protein:** 21g

Chapter 3:

Poultry Recipes

17. Cheesy Turkey Burgers

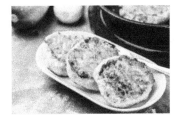

Preparation time: 10 minutes.

Cooking time: 25 minutes.

Servings: 4

Ingredients

- 2 medium yellow onions

- 1 tablespoon olive oil

- 1(½) teaspoon kosher salt, divided

- 1(¼) pound (567 grams) ground turkey

- 1/3 cup mayonnaise

- 1 tablespoon Dijon mustard

- 2 teaspoons Worcestershire sauce

- 4 slices sharp Cheddar cheese (113 grams in total)

- 4 hamburger buns, sliced

Directions:

1. Trim the onions and cut them in half through the root. Cut one of the halves in half. Grate one quarter. Place the grated onion in a large bowl. Thinly slice the remaining onions and place in a medium bowl with the oil and ½ teaspoon of kosher salt. Toss to coat. Spread the onions in a single layer on a baking pan.

2. Slide the pan into the Air Fryer oven. Press the Power Button. Cook at 350°F (180°C) for 10 minutes.

3. While the onions are cooking, add the turkey to the grated onion. Stir in the remaining kosher salt, mayonnaise, mustard, and Worcestershire sauce. Divide the mixture into 4 patties, each about ¾-inch thick.

4. When cooking is completed, remove from the Air Fryer oven. Move the onions to one side of the pan and place the burgers on the pan. Poke your finger into the center of each burger to make a deep indentation.

5. Slide the pan into the Air Fryer oven. Cook for 12 minutes.

6. After 6 minutes, remove the pan. Turn the burgers and stir the onions. Return to the Air Fryer oven and continue cooking. After about 4 minutes, remove the pan and place the cheese slices on the burgers. Return to the Air Fryer oven and continue cooking for about 1 minute, or until the cheese is melted and the center of the burgers has reached at least 165°F (74°C) on a meat thermometer.

7. When cooking is completed, remove from the Air Fryer oven. Loosely cover the burgers with foil.

8. Layout the buns, cut-side up, on the airflow racks. Cook for 3 minutes. Check the buns after 2 minutes; they should be lightly browned.

9. Remove the buns from the Air Fryer oven. Assemble the burgers and serve.

Nutrition

- **Calories:** 161

- **Protein:** 22g

- **Fat:** 18g

18. Chicken and Ham Meatballs with Dijon Sauce

Preparation time: 10 minutes.

Cooking time: 15 minutes.**Servings:** 4

Ingredients

Meatballs:

- ½ pound (227 grams) ham, diced

- ½ pound (227 grams) ground chicken

- ½ cup grated Swiss cheese

- 1 large egg, beaten

- 3 garlic cloves, minced

- ¼ cup chopped onions

- 1(½) teaspoon sea salt

- 1 teaspoon ground black pepper

- Cooking spray for greasing

Dijon Sauce:

- 3 tablespoons Dijon mustard

- 2 tablespoons lemon juice

- ¼ cup chicken broth, warmed

- ¾ teaspoon sea salt

- ¼ teaspoon ground black pepper

- Chopped fresh thyme leaves, for garnish

Directions:

1. Spray the airflow racks with cooking spray.

2. Incorporate the ingredients for the meatballs in a large bowl. Stir to mix well, then shape the mixture in twelve 1½-inch meatballs.

3. Arrange the meatballs in the airflow racks.

4. Slide the racks into the Air Fryer oven. Press the Power Button. Cook at 390°F (199°C) for 15 minutes.

5. Flip the balls halfway through.

6. When cooking is completed, the balls should be lightly browned.

7. Meanwhile, combine the ingredients, except for the thyme leaves, for the sauce in a small bowl. Stir to mix well.

8. Transfer the cooked meatballs to a large plate, then baste the sauce over. Garnish with thyme leaves and serve.

Nutrition

- **Calories:** 170

- **Protein:** 21g

- **Fat:** 14g

19. Chicken Schnitzel

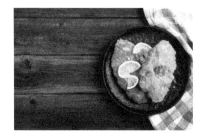

Preparation time: 15 minutes.

Cooking time: 5 minutes. **Servings:** 4

Ingredients:

- ½ cup all-purpose flour

- 1 teaspoon marjoram

- ½ teaspoon thyme

- 1 teaspoon dried parsley flakes

- ½ teaspoon salt

- 1 egg

- 1 teaspoon lemon juice

- 1 teaspoon water

- 1 cup breadcrumbs

- 4 chicken tenders, pounded thin, cut in half lengthwise

- Cooking spray for greasing

Directions:

1. Spray the airflow racks with cooking spray.

2. Combine the flour, marjoram, thyme, parsley, and salt in a shallow dish. Stir to mix well.

3. Whisk the egg with lemon juice and water in a large bowl. Pour the breadcrumbs into a separate shallow dish. Roll the chicken halves in the flour mixture first, then in the egg mixture, and then roll over the breadcrumbs to coat well. Shake the excess off.

4. Arrange the chicken halves in the airflow racks and spray with cooking spray on both sides.

5. Slide the racks into the Air Fryer oven. Press the Power Button. Cook at 390°F (199°C) for 5 minutes. Flip the halves halfway through.

6. When cooking is completed, the chicken halves should be golden brown and crispy.

7. Serve immediately.

Nutrition

- **Calories:** 133 **Protein:** 19g **Fat:** 12g

20. Chicken Shawarma

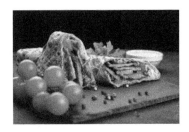

Preparation time: 10 minutes.

Cooking time: 18 minutes. **Servings:** 4

Ingredients:

- 1(½) pound (680 grams) chicken thighs

- 1(¼) teaspoon kosher salt, divided

- 2 tablespoons plus 1 teaspoon olive oil, divided

- 2/3 cup plus 2 tablespoons plain Greek yogurt, divided

- 2 tablespoons freshly squeezed lemon juice (about 1 medium

  lemon)

- 4 garlic cloves, minced, divided

- 1 tablespoon Shawarma seasoning

- 4 pita breads, cut in half

- 2 cups cherry tomatoes

- ½ small cucumber, peeled, deseeded, and chopped

- 1 tablespoon chopped fresh parsley

Directions:

1. Season the chicken thighs on both sides with 1 teaspoon of kosher salt. Place in a resealable plastic bag and set aside while you make the marinade.

2. In a small bowl, mix 2 tablespoons of olive oil, 2 tablespoons of yogurt, lemon juice, 3 garlic cloves, and Shawarma seasoning until thoroughly combined. Pour the marinade over the chicken. Wrap the bag, squeezing out as much air as possible. And massage the chicken to coat it with the sauce. Set aside.

3. Wrap 2 pita breads each in two pieces of aluminum foil and place on a baking pan.

4. Slide the pan into the Air Fryer oven. Press the power button. Cook at 300°F (150°C) for 6 minutes. After 3 minutes, remove from the Air Fryer oven and turn over the foil packets. Return to the Air Fryer oven and continue cooking. When cooking is completed, remove from the Air Fryer oven and place the foil-wrapped pitas on the top of the Air Fryer oven to keep warm.

5. Pull out the chicken from the marinade, letting the excess drip off into the bag. Place them on the baking pan. Arrange the tomatoes around the sides of the chicken. Discard the marinade.

6. Slide the pan into the Air Fryer oven. Cook for 12 minutes.

7. After 6 minutes, remove from the Air Fryer oven and turn over the chicken. Return to the Air Fryer oven and continue cooking.

8. Wrap the cucumber in a paper towel to remove as much moisture as possible. Place them in a small bowl. Add the remaining yogurt, kosher salt, olive oil, garlic clove, and parsley. Whisk until combined.

9. Pull out the pan from the Air Fryer oven and place the chicken on a cutting board. Cut each thigh into several pieces. Unwrap the pitas. Spread a tablespoon of sauce into a pita half. Add some chicken and add 2 roasted tomatoes. Serve.

Nutrition:

- **Calories:** 199

- **Protein:** 22g

- **Fat:** 6g

21. Chicken Skewers with Corn Salad

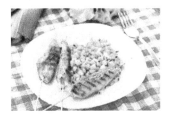

Preparation time: 17 minutes.

Cooking time: 10 minutes. **Servings:** 4

Ingredients:

- 1 pound (454 grams) chicken breast, cut into 1½-inch chunks

- 1 green bell pepper, deseeded and cut into 1-inch pieces

- 1 red bell pepper, deseeded and cut into 1-inch pieces

- 1 large onion, cut into large chunks

- 2 tablespoons fajita seasoning

- 3 tablespoons vegetable oil, divided

- 2 teaspoons kosher salt, divided

- 2 cups corn, drained

- ¼ teaspoon granulated garlic

- 1 teaspoon freshly squeezed lime juice

- 1 tablespoon mayonnaise

- 3 tablespoons grated Parmesan cheese

Directions:

1. Place the chicken, bell peppers, and onion in a large bowl. Add the fajita seasoning, 2 tablespoons of vegetable oil, and 1(½) teaspoon of kosher salt. Toss to coat evenly.

2. Alternate the chicken and vegetables on the skewers, making about 12 skewers.

3. Place the corn in a medium bowl and add the remaining vegetable oil. Add the remaining kosher salt and the garlic, and toss to coat. Place the corn in an even layer on a baking pan and place the skewers on top.

4. Slide the pan into the Air Fryer oven. Press the power button. Cook at 375°F (190°C) for 10 minutes.

5. After about 5 minutes, remove from the Air Fryer oven and turn the skewers. Return to the Air Fryer oven and continue cooking.

6. When cooking is completed, remove from the Air Fryer oven. Place the skewers on a platter. Put the corn back to the bowl and combine it with lime juice, mayonnaise, and Parmesan cheese. Stir to mix well. Serve the skewers with the corn.

Nutrition

- **Calories:** 166

- **Protein:** 17g

- **Fat:** 11g

22. Chicken Thighs in Waffles

Preparation time: 1 hour and 20 minutes.

Cooking time: 20 minutes.

Servings: 4

Ingredients:

For the chicken:

- 4 chicken thighs, skin on

- 1 cup low-fat buttermilk

- ½ cup all-purpose flour

- ½ teaspoon garlic powder

- ½ teaspoon mustard powder

- 1 teaspoon kosher salt

- ½ teaspoon freshly ground black pepper

- ¼ cup honey, for serving

- Cooking spray for greasing

For the waffles:

- ½ cup all-purpose flour

- ½ cup whole wheat pastry flour

- 1 large egg, beaten

- 1 cup low-fat buttermilk

- 1 teaspoon baking powder

- 2 tablespoons canola oil

- ½ teaspoon kosher salt

- 1 tablespoon granulated sugar

Directions:

1. Combine the chicken thighs with buttermilk in a large bowl. Wrap the bowl in plastic and refrigerate to marinate for at least an hour.

2. Spray the airflow racks with cooking spray.

3. Combine the flour, mustard powder, garlic powder, salt, and black pepper in a shallow dish. Stir to mix well.

4. Remove the thighs from the buttermilk and pat dry with paper towels. Sit the bowl of buttermilk aside.

5. Dip the thighs in the flour mixture first, then into the buttermilk, and then into the flour mixture. Shake the excess off.

6. Arrange the thighs in the airflow racks and spray with cooking spray.

7. Slide the racks into the Air Fryer oven. Press the Power Button. Cook at 360°F (182°C) for 20 minutes.

8. Flip the thighs halfway through.

9. When cooking is completed, an instant-read thermometer inserted in the thickest part of the chicken thighs should register at least 165°F (74°C).

10. Meanwhile, make the waffles: combine the ingredients for the waffles in a large bowl. Stir to mix well, then arrange the mixture in a waffle iron and cook until a golden and fragrant waffle is formed.

11. Remove the waffles from the waffle iron and slice into 4 pieces. Remove the chicken thighs from the Air Fryer oven and allow cooling for 5 minutes.

12. Arrange each chicken thigh on each waffle piece and drizzle with 1 tablespoon of honey. Serve warm.

Nutrition

- **Calories:** 188

- **Protein:** 21g

- **Fat:** 9g

Chapter 4:

Vegetables Recipes

23. Healthy Artichoke Casserole

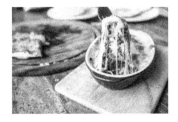

Preparation time: 10 minutes.

Cooking time: 30 minutes.

Servings: 12

Ingredients:

- 16 eggs

- 14 ounces can artichoke hearts, drained and cut into pieces

- 1/4 cup coconut milk

- 1/2 teaspoon red pepper, crushed

- 1/2 teaspoon thyme, diced

- 1/2 cup ricotta cheese

- 1/2 cup Parmesan cheese

- 1 cup Cheddar cheese, shredded

- 10 ounces frozen spinach, thawed and drain well

- 1 garlic clove, minced

- 1/4 cup onion, shaved

- 1 teaspoon salt

Directions:

1. In a large bowl, whisk together eggs and coconut milk.

2. Add spinach and artichoke into the egg mixture.

3. Add all the remaining ingredients, except for ricotta cheese and

   stir well to combine.

4. Place the inner pot in the Power grill Air Fryer combo base.

5. Pour egg mixture into the inner pot.

6. Spread ricotta cheese on top of the egg mixture.

7. Cover the inner pot with an air frying lid.

8. Select bake mode,then set the temperature to 350°F and time for 30 minutes. Click start.

9. When the timer reaches 0, then press the cancel button.

10. Serve and enjoy!

Nutrition:

- **Calories:** 205

- **Fat:** 13.7g

- **Protein:** 15.9g

24. Baked Tomato

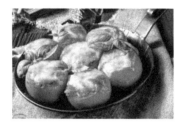

Preparation time: 10 minutes.

Cooking time: 30 minutes.

Servings: 2

Ingredients:

- 2 eggs

- 2 large fresh tomatoes

- 1 teaspoon fresh parsley

- Pepper to taste

- Salt to taste

Directions:

1. Cut off the top of a tomato and spoon out the tomato innards.

2. Break the egg in each tomato.

3. Place the inner pot in the Power grill Air Fryer combo base.

4. Place tomato into the inner pot.

5. Cover the inner pot with an air frying lid.

6. Select bake mode, then set the temperature to 350°F and time for 15 minutes. Click start.

7. When the timer reaches 0, then press the cancel button.

8. Season tomato with parsley, pepper, and salt.

9. Serve and enjoy!

Nutrition:

- **Calories:** 96

- **Fat:** 4.7g

- **Protein:** 7.2g

25. Baked Cauliflower

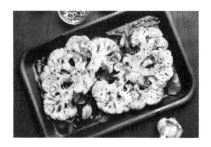

Preparation time: 10 minutes.

Cooking time: 45 minutes. **Servings:** 2

Ingredients:

- 1/2 cauliflower head, cut into florets

- 2 tablespoons olive oil

For seasoning:

- 1/2 teaspoon white pepper

- 1/2 teaspoon garlic powder

- 1/2 teaspoon ground cumin

- 1/2 teaspoon black pepper

- 1/2 teaspoon ground cayenne

- 1 teaspoon onion powder

- 1/4 teaspoon dried oregano

- 1/4 teaspoon dried basil

- 1/4 teaspoon dried thyme

- 1/4 tablespoon ground paprika

- ¼ teaspoon salt

Directions:

1. In a large bowl, mix together all seasoning ingredients.

2. Add oil and stir well. Add cauliflower to the bowl, seasoning mixture, and stir well to coat.

3. Place the inner pot in the Power grill Air Fryer combo base.

4. Spread the cauliflower florets into the inner pot.

5. Cover the inner pot with an air frying lid.

6. Select bake mode, then set the temperature to 400°F and time for 45 minutes. Click start.

7. When the timer reaches 0, then press the cancel button.

8. Serve and enjoy!

Nutrition:

- **Calories:** 177

- **Fat:** 15.6g

- **Protein:** 3.1g

26. Easy Baked Beans

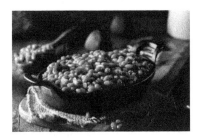

Preparation time: 10 minutes.

Cooking time: 10 minutes.

Servings: 2

Ingredients:

- 16 ounces can white beans, drained and rinsed

- 2 tablespoons BBQ sauce

- 1(1/2) tablespoon maple syrup

- 1(1/2) teaspoon lemon juice

- 1 tablespoon prepared yellow mustard

Directions:

1. Place the inner pot in the Power grill Air Fryer combo base.

2. Add all the ingredients into the inner pot and stir well.

3. Cover the inner pot with a glass lid.

4. Select simmer mode, then presses the temperature button and set the time for 10 minutes. Click start.

5. When the timer reaches 0, then press the cancel button.

6. Stir well and serve.

Nutrition:

- **Calories:** 278

- **Fat:** 0.4g

- **Protein:** 14g

27. Creamy Cauliflower Casserole

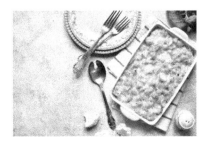

Preparation time: 10 minutes.

Cooking time: 15 minutes.

Servings: 6

Ingredients:

- 1 cauliflower head, cut into florets, and boil

- 2 cups Cheddar cheese, shredded

- 2 teaspoons Dijon mustard

- 2 ounces cream cheese

- 1 cup heavy cream

- 1 teaspoon garlic powder

- 1/2 teaspoon pepper

- 1/2 teaspoon salt

Directions:

1. Place the inner pot in the Power grill Air Fryer combo base.

2. Add all the ingredients into the inner pot and mix well.

3. Cover the inner pot with an air frying lid.

4. Select bake mode, then set the temperature to 375°F and time for 15 minutes. Click start.

5. When the timer reaches 0, then press the cancel button.

6. Serve and enjoy!

Nutrition:

- **Calories:** 268

- **Fat:** 23.3g

- **Protein:** 11.5g

28. Baked Eggplant & Zucchini

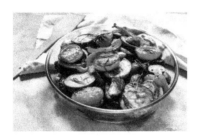

Preparation time: 10 minutes.

Cooking time: 35 minutes. **Servings:** 6

Ingredients:

- 1 medium eggplant, sliced

- 3 medium zucchinis, sliced

- 3 ounces Parmesan cheese, grated

- 4 tablespoons parsley, chopped

- 4 tablespoons basil, chopped

- 1 tablespoon olive oil

- 4 garlic cloves, minced

- 1 cup cherry tomatoes, halved

- 1/4 teaspoon pepper

- 1/4 teaspoon salt

Directions:

1. In a mixing bowl, add cherry tomatoes, eggplant, zucchini, olive oil, garlic, cheese, basil, pepper, and salt toss well until combined.

2. Transfer the eggplant mixture into the greased baking dish.

3. Place the inner pot in the Power grill Air Fryer combo base.

4. Place baking dish into the inner pot. Cover the inner pot with an air frying lid.

5. Select bake mode, then set the temperature to 350°F and time for 35 minutes. Click start.

6. When the timer reaches 0, then press the cancel button.

7. Garnish with chopped parsley and serve.

Nutrition:

- **Calories:** 110 **Fat:** 5.8g **Protein:** 7.0g

29. Scalloped Potatoes

Preparation time: 10 minutes.

Cooking time: 45 minutes.

Servings: 6

Ingredients:

- 4 sweet potatoes, peeled

- 1/4 cup olive oil

- 1/2 teaspoon paprika

- 1 tablespoon maple syrup

- 1/2 cup fresh orange juice

- 1/2 teaspoon orange zest

- 1 teaspoon salt

Directions:

1. Slice sweet potatoes 1/16-inch thick using a slicer.

2. Arrange sweet potato slices into the greased baking dish.

3. In a bowl, whisk together the remaining ingredients and pour over sweet potatoes.

4. Place the inner pot in the Power grill Air Fryer combo base.

5. Place baking dish into the inner pot.

6. Cover the inner pot with an air frying lid.

7. Select bake mode, then set the temperature to 350°F and time for 45 minutes. Click start.

8. When the timer reaches 0, then press the cancel button.

9. Serve and enjoy!

Nutrition:

- **Calories:** 91

- **Fat:** 8.6g

- **Protein:** 1.7g

30. Healthy Broccoli Casserole

Preparation time: 10 minutes.

Cooking time: 30 minutes.

Servings: 6

Ingredients:

- 15 ounces broccoli florets

- 10 ounces can cream of mushroom soup

- 1 cup mozzarella cheese, shredded

- 1/3 cup milk

- 1/2 teaspoon onion powder

For topping:

- 1 tablespoon butter, melted

- 1/2 cup crushed crackers

Directions:

1. Place the inner pot in the Power grill Air Fryer combo base.

2. Add all the ingredients, except for the topping ingredients into the inner pot.

3. In a small bowl, mix together cracker crumbs and melted butter and sprinkle over the inner pot mixture.

4. Cover the inner pot with an air frying lid.

5. Select bake mode, then set the temperature to 350°F and time for 30 minutes. Click start.

6. When the timer reaches 0, then press the cancel button.

7. Serve and enjoy!

Nutrition:

- **Calories:** 179

- **Fat:** 10.6g

- **Protein:** 7g

31. Thai Spicy Napa Vegetables

Preparation time: 10 minutes. **Cooking time:** 8 minutes.

Servings: 4

Ingredients:

- 1 Small head Napa cabbage, shredded, divided

- 1 medium carrot, cut into thin coins

- 8 ounces (227 grams) snow peas

- 1 red or green bell pepper, sliced into thin strips

- 1 tablespoon vegetable oil 3 tablespoons soy sauce

- 1 tablespoon sesame oil 2 tablespoons brown sugar

- 2 tablespoons freshly squeezed lime juice

- 2 teaspoons red or green Thai curry paste

- 1 serrano chili, deseeded and minced

- 1 cup frozen mango slices, thawed

- ½ cup chopped Toasted peanuts or cashews

Directions:

1. Put half the Napa cabbage in a large bowl, along with the carrot, bell pepper, and snow peas. Drizzle with the vegetable oil and toss to coat. Spread them evenly on the sheet pan.

2. Place the pan in the toast position.

3. Select Toast, set temperature to 375°F (190°C), and set time to 8 minutes.

4. Meanwhile, whisk together the soy sauce, brown sugar, sesame oil, curry paste, and lime juice in a small bowl.

5. When done, the vegetables should be tender and crisp. Remove the pan and put the vegetables back into the bowl. Add the remaining cabbage, mango slices, and chile. Pour over the dressing and toss to coat. Top with the toasted nuts and serve.

Nutrition:

- **Calories:** 810 **Fat:** 23g **Protein:** 68g

Chapter 5:

Fish and Seafood Recipes

32. Crispy Halibut Fillets

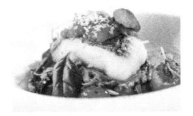

Preparation time: 5 minutes.

Cooking time: 9 minutes.

Servings: 4

Ingredients:

- 2 medium-sized halibut fillets

- A dash of tabasco sauce

- ½ teaspoon curry powder

- ½ teaspoon ground coriander

- ½ teaspoon hot paprika

- Kosher salt and freshly cracked mixed peppercorns to taste

- 2 eggs

- ½ cup grated Parmesan cheese

- 1(½) tablespoons olive oil

Directions:

1. On a clean work surface, drizzle the halibut fillets with the tabasco sauce. Sprinkle with curry powder, hot paprika, coriander, salt, and cracked mixed peppercorns. Set aside.

2. In a shallow bowl, beat the eggs until frothy. In another shallow bowl, combine the Parmesan cheese and olive oil.

3. One at a time, dredge the halibut fillets in the beaten eggs, shaking off any excess, then roll them over the Parmesan cheese until evenly coated.

4. Arrange the halibut fillets in the Air Fry basket in a single layer.

5. Place the basket in the Toast position.

6. Select Toast, set temperature to 365°F (185°C), and set time to 10 minutes.

7. When cooking is completed, the fish should be golden brown and crisp. Cool for 5 minutes before serving.

Nutrition:

- **Calories:** 864

- **Fat:** 32g

- **Protein:** 63g

33. Salmon Fillet with Tomatoes

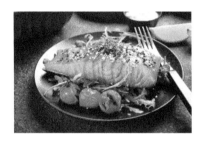

Preparation time: 10 minutes

Cooking time: 16 minutes **Servings:** 4

Ingredients:

- 4(6-ounces) salmon fillets, patted dry

- 1 teaspoon kosher salt, divided

- 2 cups (1 pint) cherry or grape tomatoes, halved if large, divided

- 3 tablespoons extra-virgin olive oil, divided

- 2 garlic cloves, minced 1 small red bell pepper, deseeded and

  chopped 2 tablespoons chopped fresh basil, divided

Directions:

1. Season both sides of the salmon with ½ teaspoon of kosher salt.

2. Put about half of the tomatoes in a large bowl, along with 2 tablespoons of olive oil, the remaining ½ teaspoon of kosher salt, bell pepper, garlic, and 1 tablespoon of basil. Toss to coat and then transfer to the sheet pan.

3. Arrange the salmon fillets on the sheet pan, skin-side down. Brush them with the remaining 1 tablespoon of olive oil.

4. Place the pan in the Toast position.

5. Select Toast, set temperature to 375°F (190°C), and set time to 15 minutes.

6. After 7 minutes, remove the pan and fold in the remaining tomatoes. Return the pan to the Air Fryer grill and continue cooking.

7. When cooked, remove the pan from the Air Fryer grill. Serve sprinkled with the remaining 1 tablespoon of basil.

Nutrition:

*   **Calories:** 774 **Fat:** 37g **Protein:** 77g

34. Teriyaki Salmon with Bok Choy

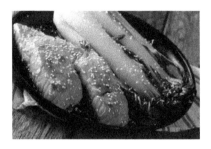

Preparation time: 15 minutes.

Cooking time: 15 minutes. **Servings:** 4

Ingredients:

- ¾ cup Teriyaki sauce, divided 4 (6-ounces/170 grams) skinless salmon fillets 4 heads baby bok choy, root ends trimmed off and cut in half lengthwise through the root

- 1 teaspoon sesame oil 1 tablespoon vegetable oil

- 1 tablespoon toasted sesame seeds

Directions:

1. Set aside ¼ cup of Teriyaki sauce and pour the remaining sauce into a resealable plastic bag. Put the salmon into the bag and seal,

squeezing as much air out as possible. Allow the salmon to marinate for at least 10 minutes.

2. Arrange the bok choy halves on the sheet pan. Drizzle the oils over the vegetables, tossing to coat. Drizzle about 1 tablespoon of the reserved teriyaki sauce over the bok choy, then push them to the sides of the sheet pan.

3. Put the salmon fillets in the middle of the sheet pan.

4. Place the pan in the Toast position.

5. Select toast, set temperature to 375°F (190°C), and set time to 15 minutes.

6. When done, remove the pan and brush the salmon with the remaining teriyaki sauce. Serve garnished with sesame seeds.

Nutrition:

*   **Calories:** 624 **Fat:** 21g

*   **Protein:** 68g

35. Golden Fish Fillets

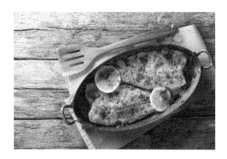

Preparation time: 20 minutes.

Cooking time: 9 minutes. **Servings:** 4

Ingredients:

- ½ pound fish fillets

- 1 tablespoon coarse brown mustard

- 1 teaspoon Worcestershire sauce

- ½ teaspoon hot sauce - Salt to taste

- Cooking spray for greasing

Crumb coating:

- ¾ cup panko breadcrumbs

- ¼ cup stone-ground cornmeal

- ¼ teaspoon salt

Directions:

1. On your cutting board, cut the fish fillets crosswise into slices, about 1 inch wide.

2. In a small bowl, stir together the Worcestershire sauce, mustard, and hot sauce to make a paste and rub this paste on all sides of the fillets. Season with salt to taste.

3. In a shallow bowl, thoroughly combine all the ingredients for the crumb coating and spread them on a sheet of wax paper. Roll the fish fillets in the crumb mixture until thickly coated. Spray all sides of the fish with cooking spray, then arrange them in the air fry basket in a single layer. Place the Air Fry basket into the Air Fryer grill.

4. Select Air Fry, set temperature to 400°F (205°C), and set time to 7 minutes.

5. When cooking is completed, the fish should flake apart with a

   fork. Remove from the Air Fryer grill and serve warm.

Nutrition:

- **Calories:** 624 **Fat:** 48g **Protein:** 99g

36. Crispy Paprika Fish Fillets

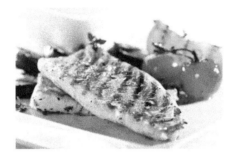

Preparation time: 5 minutes.

Cooking time: 19 minutes.

Servings: 4

Ingredients:

- 1/2 cup seasoned breadcrumbs

- 1 tablespoon balsamic vinegar

- 1/2 teaspoon seasoned salt

- 1 teaspoon paprika

- 1/2 teaspoon ground black pepper

- 1 teaspoon celery seed

- 2 fish fillets, halved

- 1 egg, beaten

Directions:

1. Add the breadcrumbs, vinegar, salt, paprika, ground black pepper, and celery seeds to your food processor. Process for about 30 seconds.

2. Coat the fish fillets with the beaten egg; then, coat them with the breadcrumb's mixture.

3. Cook at 350°F for about 15 minutes.

Nutrition:

- **Calories:** 884

- **Fat:** 43g

- **Protein:** 80g

37. Crispy Cheesy Fish Fingers

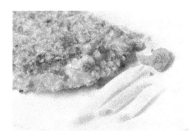

Preparation time: 10 minutes.

Cooking time: 19 minutes. **Servings:** 4

Ingredients:

- 6–8 ounces large codfish filet, fresh or frozen, cut into 1 ½-inch

  strip

- 2 raw eggs

- ½ cup of breadcrumbs (we like Panko, but any brand or home

  recipe will do)

- 2 tablespoons of shredded or powdered Parmesan cheese

- 3 tablespoons of shredded Cheddar cheese

- Pinch of salt and pepper

Directions:

1. Cover the basket of the XL Air Fryer oven with a lining of tin foil, leaving the edges uncovered to allow air to circulate through the basket. Preheat the Air Fryer oven to 350°F.

2. In a large mixing bowl, beat the eggs until fluffy and until the yolks and whites are fully combined. Dunk all the fish strips in the beaten eggs, fully submerging.

3. In a separate mixing bowl, combine the breadcrumbs with the Parmesan, Cheddar, and salt and pepper, until evenly mixed.

4. One by one, coat the egg-covered fish strips in the mixed dry ingredients so that they're fully covered, and place them on the foil-lined oven rack/basket. Place the rack on the middle-shelf of the XL Air Fryer oven. Set the air-fryer timer to 20 minutes.

5. Halfway through the cooking time, shake the handle of the air-fryer so that the breaded fish jostles inside and fry-coverage is even.

6. After 20 minutes, when the fryer shuts off, the fish strips will be perfectly cooked and their breaded crust golden-brown and delicious! Using tongs, remove from the Air Fryer oven and place on a serving dish to cool.

Nutrition:

- **Calories:** 814 **Fat:** 31g **Protein:** 71g

38. Panko-Crusted Tilapia

Preparation time: 5 minutes.

Cooking time: 10 minutes.

Servings: 3

Ingredients:

- 2 teaspoons Italian seasoning

- 2 teaspoons lemon pepper

- 1/3 cup panko breadcrumbs

- 1/3 cup egg whites

- 1/3 cup almond flour

- 3 tilapia fillets

- Olive oil for greasing

Directions:

1. Place panko, egg whites, and flour into separate bowls. Mix lemon pepper and Italian seasoning with breadcrumbs.

2. Pat tilapia fillets dry. Dredge in flour, egg, and breadcrumb mixture.

3. Add to the oven rack/basket and spray lightly with olive oil. Place the rack on the middle-shelf of the XL Air Fryer oven.

4. Cook 10–11 minutes at 400°F, making sure to flip halfway through cooking.

Nutrition:

- **Calories:** 256

- **Fat:** 9g

- **Protein:** 39g

Chapter 6:

Snacks Recipes

39. Shrimp Bacon Bites

Preparation time: 8 to 10 minutes.

Cooking time: 8 minutes.

Servings: 8 to 10

Ingredients:

- 1/2 teaspoon red pepper flakes, crushed

- 1 tablespoon salt

- 1 teaspoon chili powder

- 1 ¼ pounds shrimp, peeled and deveined

- 1 teaspoon paprika

- 1/2 teaspoon black pepper, ground

- 1 tablespoon shallot powder

- 1/4 teaspoon cumin powder

- 1 ¼ pounds thin bacon slices

Directions:

1. Place your Air Fryer on a flat kitchen surface; plug it and turn it on. Set temperature to 360°F and let it preheat for 4–5 minutes.

2. Take out the Air-frying basket and gently coat it using cooking oil or spray.

3. In a bowl of medium size, thoroughly mix the shrimp and seasoning until they are coated well.

4. Now wrap a slice of bacon around the shrimps; secure them with a toothpick and refrigerate for 30 minutes.

5. Add the shrimps to the basket. Push the Air-frying basket in the Air Fryer. Cook for 8 minutes.

6. Slide-out the basket; serve with cocktail sticks or your choice of dip (optional).

Nutrition:

- **Calories:** 374

- **Fat:** 28.2g

- **Carbohydrates:** 2g

- **Fiber:** 0g

- **Protein:** 34.3g

Chapter 7:

Desserts Recipes

40. Roasted Bananas

Preparation time: 5 minutes.

Cooking time: 5 minutes.

Servings: 2

Ingredients:

- 2 cups bananas, cubed

- 1 teaspoon avocado oil

- 1 tablespoon maple syrup

- 1 teaspoon brown sugar

- 1 cup almond milk

Directions:

1. Coat the banana cubes with oil and maple syrup.

2. Sprinkle with brown sugar.

3. Cook at 375°F in the Air Fryer for 5 minutes.

4. Drizzle milk on top of the bananas before serving.

Nutrition:

- **Calories:** 107

- **Protein:** 1.3g

- **Fat:** 0.7g

- **Carbs:** 27g

Conclusion

Air frying your food is one of the great alternative methods of deep-frying your food. There are various advanced Air Fryers available on the market now. In this cookbook, we have used such smart, advanced, and multifunctional cooking appliances popularly known as Power Air Fryer oven. The Power oven allows you to cook almost all types of dishes in a single cooking appliance. It is capable to cook vegetables, meat, fish, fruit slices, cakes, and more. The oven comes with different accessories, using these accessories you can cook a healthy and delicious meal at home easily. The oven is capable of roasting whole turkey or chicken at a single cooking cycle.

The Power Air Fryer is an effortless way to cook healthy and delicious foods. As a replacement for using oil, this one uses air to cook. You can cook all sorts of food, even appetizers, and snacks. Foods are cooked fast and evenly without oils. Relish cooking healthier than ever before.

The Power Air Fryer oven works on a rapid hot airflow technique which helps to distribute equally the heat into the cooking chamber around the food. This equal heat distribution cooks your food faster and gives you even cooking results in every cooking cycle. It makes your food crispy from the outside, juicy and tender from the inside. The oven comes with a big display panel with 8 preset functions. While using these preset functions, you will never be worried about temperature and time settings, as they are preset. You can also set these settings manually by pressing the up and down arrow key, pressing the up and down arrow keys given on the control panel.

This amazing appliance is simple to use. Just add the food you wish to cook and turn the 3 burners on. You can grill, fry, roast, bake, and even smoke. It can also be used to steam, boil, dehydrate and freeze. Using the Complete Power fryer, there are no limitations on what you can cook. You can also easily make healthy takeout food that would cost you a fortune.

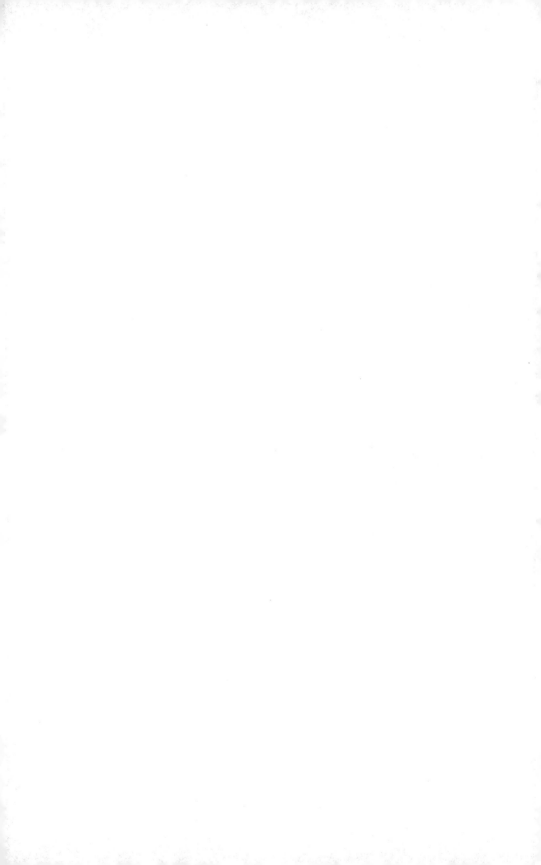